The Role of Diet in Diabetes Management:

Debunking Myths and Embracing Evidence-Based Nutrition

By

Dr. Emily Collins

Copyright © 2024

Disclaimer

This book's content on health improvement is meant only for general educational purposes. It is not intended to replace expert medical guidance, diagnosis, or care. Before modifying their diet, exercise routine, or way of life, readers should speak with a licensed healthcare provider. The use of the information in this book may have unintended effects, for which the author and publisher disclaim all liability.

About the Author

Introducing Dr. Emily Collins: Advancing the Conversation on Nutrition and Diabetes The pioneering conversation on dietary treatments in diabetes care is led by the esteemed physician and researcher, Dr. Emily Collins. Her landmark book, "The Role of Diet in Diabetes Management," is more than simply a book; for millions of people struggling with this widespread metabolic illness, it is a manifesto of hope. Dr. Collins was a trailblazer from the beginning, motivated by a strong desire to understand the complex relationship between diabetes and diet. Her path was profoundly personal in addition to being academic. Seeing the difficulties her own family faced with diabetes sparked a desire to solve the puzzles around food habits and how they affect blood sugar regulation.Through countless hours of study and clinical work, Dr. Collins cleared the way for people with diabetes to take charge of their own care. Her book offers approachable ideas and useful solutions for negotiating the challenging landscape of dietary choices, going beyond the bounds of conventional medical literature. With relentless commitment, Dr. Collins broke down stereotypes, questioned established wisdom, and led the way in a paradigm shift in the treatment of diabetes. She promoted a comprehensive strategy that included customized nutrition regimens based on each patient's particular metabolic profile and way of life. "The Role of Diet in Diabetes Management" inspires people to take back control of their health outcomes by serving as a beacon of empowerment rather than just a compilation of scientific research findings. The impact of Dr. Collins' work extends beyond academic circles, touching patients, caregivers, and medical professionals in equal measure.Dr. Emily Collins shines as a ray of hope in a world where diabetes is becoming a more pressing problem by demonstrating the transforming power of dietary treatments in the never-ending quest for health and vitality.

Table of contents

Introduction

Diabetes, a long-term metabolic disease marked by high blood sugar, is now a major global health issue that affects millions of people. Although genetic predisposition contributes, lifestyle factors especially diet have a major impact on the development and treatment of CVD. For both those who already have diabetes and those who want to avoid getting it, it is essential to comprehend the critical role that nutrition plays in managing the disease.Overview of Diabetes: An Expanding Epidemic Diabetes, often known as diabetes mellitus, is a collective term for a series of illnesses marked by elevated glucose.glucose levels brought on by deficiencies in the action or secretion of insulin, or both. Type 1 and type 2 diabetes are the two main types, and they each have different causes and courses of therapy. Usually occurring in childhood or adolescence, type 1 diabetes is caused by the immune system destroying the beta cells in the pancreas that produce insulin. For the rest of their lives, people with type 1 diabetes need to take insulin to keep their blood sugar levels within a normal range. The most common kind of diabetes, type 2, usually appears in adulthood and is strongly linked to lifestyle choices like obesity, sedentary lifestyles, and unhealthy eating patterns. Diabetes type 2 causes the body to either Hyperglycemia is caused when the body either develops resistance to insulin or is unable to produce enough of it to meet its needs. Over 400 million individuals may be affected globally, according to estimates, indicating that the prevalence of diabetes has reached frightening heights. Furthermore, there are major health risks and financial burdens associated with diabetes-related problems for both individuals and healthcare systems worldwide. These include cardiovascular disease, kidney failure, and neuropathy.

Chapter one

Understanding Diabetes

Diabetes, often known as diabetes mellitus, is a long-term metabolic disease marked by high blood glucose levels brought on by either insufficient insulin production, resistance to the effects of insulin, or both. Though it presents serious health concerns and affects millions of people globally, managing and preventing this disorder effectively requires an awareness of its complexities.

Diabetes Types

1. Diabetes Type 1: Cause: A complete lack of insulin is the outcome of type 1 diabetes, which is caused by the autoimmune death of the pancreatic beta cells that produce insulin.The condition is usually identified in childhood or adolescence, but it can manifest at any stage of life.Treatment: injectable insulin or use an insulin pump for lifetime insulin therapy.

2. Diabetes Type 2:

Etiology: Insulin resistance, or the inability of cells to respond to insulin as well as the inability of pancreatic beta cells to create enough insulin to overcome this resistance, is the root cause of type 2 diabetes.Origin: More prevalent in adults, although as obesity rates rise, children and adolescents are being diagnosed with the condition more frequently.Treatment: Injectable therapy, oral drugs, lifestyle changes, and occasionally insulin are used to manage the condition.

3. Gestational Diabetes:

Etiology: Hormonal alterations that affect insulin function during pregnancy are the cause of this condition.Risk factors include obesity or overweight, a family history of diabetes, and a history of gestational diabetes.Complications: This raises the possibility of problems for the mother and child.Management: modifications to diet, tracking of blood sugar, and occasionally insulin treatment.

Diabetes's Pathophysiology

Insulin and the Regulation of Blood Sugar:
Insulin is generated by the pancreatic beta cells and aids in the uptake of glucose into cells for the synthesis and storage of energy.
Hyperglycemia is a condition in which low insulin action raises blood glucose levels.

Important Mechanisms:
Diabetes Type 1: Insulin output is decreased when beta cells are destroyed by the immune system.

Type 2 diabetes is characterized by reduced insulin production from pancreatic beta cells and tissue insulin resistance.

Clinical Signs and Symptoms:

Typical indications consist of:
*polyuria (repeated urination)

*Overindulgence in thirst, or polydipsia

*Polyphagia, or heightened appetite

* Exhaustion

 *Loss of weight (Type 1)

 *Distorted vision

 * Sluggish healing of wounds

Complications of Diabetes:
　　1.　Immediate complications:

Hypoglycemia: low blood sugar brought on by either an insufficient or an excessive amount of insulin.

Hyperglycemia: excessive blood sugar levels that result in symptoms like weariness, increased thirst, and frequent urination.

　　2.　Long-term complications include peripheral vascular disease, coronary artery disease, and stroke.

　　　*Macrovascular complications include cardiovascular diseases.

*Microvascular complications: which impact
the kidneys, nerves, and eyes, respectively, as
retinopathy, nephropathy, and neuropathy.

Identification and Tracking:
The following tests are diagnostic:

*Fasting Plasma Glucose (FPG) TestThe OGTT.

*Oral glucose tolerance test.

*Test for hemoglobin A1c (HbA1c).

Monitoring parameters:
checking blood sugar levels with glucometers.
HbA1c values show the average blood sugar levels
for the previous two to three months.

Techniques of Management:
Changes in Lifestyle:

A nutritious diet should focus on whole grains,
fruits, vegetables, lean meats, and minimal amounts
of sugar and saturated fats.

Frequent exercise improves sensitivity to insulin and helps control weight.

Medication:

 *Oral Antidiabetic Drugs: SGLT2 inhibitors, DPP-4 inhibitors, sulfonylureas, metformin, etc.

  *Injectable treatments: GLP-1 receptor agonists and insulin.

With continuous glucose monitoring (CGM), you can improve your glycemic management by receiving real-time glucose levels and warnings.

Strategies for Prevention:

Primary prevention: adopt a healthy lifestyle with a balanced diet, frequent exercise, and weight control.
The early diagnosis and treatment of prediabetes.

Secondary Prevention: Frequent examination for complications and risk factors related to diabetes. Assistance and education to help people with diabetes take good care of their illness.

Chapter two

The Link Between Diet and Diabetes

Chronic metabolic disorders like diabetes, which impact millions of people worldwide and heavily tax healthcare systems, have reached epidemic proportions. Diabetes is influenced by genetics and lifestyle choices, but nutrition is a key element in the illness's development, treatment, and prevention. To improve health outcomes and lessen the effects of diabetes on people and societies, it is crucial to comprehend the complex interaction between nutrition and the illness.

Diabetes: What Is It?

A collection of metabolic diseases, often referred to as diabetes mellitus, are marked by increased blood glucose levels, which can be caused by abnormalities in insulin action, production, or both. Type 1 and type 2, the two main types of diabetes, have different etiologies and clinical manifestations.

Insulin shortage is the outcome of the autoimmune loss of pancreatic beta cells in type 1 diabetes, which is frequently diagnosed in childhood or adolescence. On the other hand, type 2 diabetes usually appears in adulthood and is linked to insulin resistance, a condition in which cells are unable to react to the action of insulin.Effective management measures are crucial since diabetes, regardless of type, has severe health hazards such as renal failure, blindness, nerve damage, and cardiovascular disease.

The Role of Diet in Diabetes

A key component of managing diabetes is diet, which has a significant impact on insulin sensitivity, glucose metabolism, and general health. Important dietary components that affect the development and risk of diabetes are fiber content, glycemic index

(GI), macronutrient composition, and total calorie intake.

Controlling blood sugar and carbohydrates

The quantity and quality of carbohydrates have a major effect on blood glucose levels. Refined sugars and processed grains are examples of high-glycemic carbs that raise blood sugar levels quickly, taxing the body's ability to respond to insulin and raising the risk of diabetes.

On the other hand, because low-glycemic carbs are broken down more gradually, they improve glycemic control and cause blood glucose levels to rise gradually. Examples of these foods include whole grains, legumes, fruits, and vegetables. Diabetes risk can be decreased, and blood sugar levels can be stabilized, by placing an emphasis on these complex carbs in the diet.

The Importance of Fiber

Rich in fruits, vegetables, whole grains, and legumes, dietary fiber has several health advantages, especially for those who have diabetes. Fiber has three important functions for controlling diabetes: it slows the absorption of glucose, increases satiety, and helps with weight management.

Furthermore, by postponing the absorption of carbohydrates and enhancing insulin sensitivity, soluble fiber, in particular, generates a gel-like substance in the digestive tract that can help control blood sugar levels.

Considering Protein and Fat

Although blood sugar levels are significantly influenced by carbohydrates, fat and protein also play important roles in the control of diabetes. Lean protein sources, like chicken, are included in this. Legumes, seafood, and tofu can all help control blood sugar levels and increase feelings of fullness.Nuts, seeds, avocados, and olive oil are rich sources of monounsaturated and polyunsaturated fats that are good for the heart and help preserve insulin sensitivity. But moderation is the key, since consuming too much fat can lead to insulin resistance and weight gain.

Individualized Approaches to Diabetes Management

Dietary strategies that are customized to each person's needs, tastes, and metabolic profiles are necessary for the best possible control of diabetes. Although the general dietary guidelines offer a foundation for a balanced diet, people with diabetes should collaborate closely with healthcare providers, such as registered dietitians and diabetes educators, to create customized meal plans and lifestyle modifications.

The Significance of Exercise

For the control of diabetes and general health, frequent physical exercise is crucial in addition to dietary adjustments. Exercise encourages weight loss and maintenance, increases muscle uptake of glucose, and increases insulin sensitivity.

Combining resistance training with aerobic exercises like swimming, cycling, or walking can improve cardiovascular health and blood sugar regulation. Furthermore, regular exercise raises mood, lowers stress levels, and generally improves quality of life for diabetics.

The Effect of Lifestyle Decisions

Diabetes risk and outcomes are influenced by lifestyle decisions such as smoking, alcohol drinking, and stress management, in addition to nutritional components and physical exercise. It is crucial to quit smoking since smoking aggravates insulin resistance and raises the risk of cardiovascular problems in people with diabetes.

Drinking too much alcohol can cause blood sugar levels to fluctuate, impede judgment, and result in weight gain. As such, people with diabetes should exercise caution and restraint when they consume alcohol.

Chapter three

Embracing Evidence-Based Nutrition

Diabetes, a long-term metabolic disease marked by high blood sugar, is becoming a major global health issue. Its prevalence is constantly increasing globally; hence, it is essential to have good management measures. Adopting evidence-based nutrition, which includes eating habits backed by thorough scientific study, is one viable strategy for optimizing diabetes treatment and enhancing general health outcomes.

Knowing About Diabetes and How It Affects Diet

Diabetes is a broad term that includes a number of disorders, the most common of which are Type 1 and Type 2 diabetes, each with its own etiology and therapeutic strategies. Type 2 diabetes is characterized by insulin resistance and a relative insulin deficit, which are frequently impacted by lifestyle variables. Type 1 diabetes is caused by an autoimmune attack on pancreatic beta cells, which leads to insulin deficiency.

An essential component of managing diabetes is nutrition. Blood glucose levels are greatly impacted by the consumption of carbohydrates in particular; thus, moderation and careful monitoring are required. Furthermore, dietary decisions affect cardiovascular health, lipid profiles, and weight management—all crucial components of diabetes therapy.

The Transition from Theory to Evidence-Based Nutrition

In the past, dietary guidelines for managing diabetes were frequently broad and without adequate scientific support. However, improvements in nutritional science and epidemiological research have sparked a paradigm shift in favor of evidence-based nutrition in recent decades.

Research-based nutrition highlights how important it is for dietary guidelines and recommendations to be shaped by empirical research. Strict clinical trials, comprehensive reviews, and meta-analyses are used to assess the safety and effectiveness of different nutritional therapies in the context of managing diabetes.

Important Guidelines for Diabetes: Evidence-Based Nutrition

1. Individualized Approach: Evidence-based nutrition promotes individualized dietary programs catered to each patient's needs, preferences, and metabolic profile, acknowledging the variability of diabetes presentations and patient preferences.

2. Carbohydrate Management: Although they are the main energy source, carbohydrates must be carefully

monitored and moderated due to their impact on blood glucose levels. To maximize glycemic control, evidence-based nutrition highlights the significance of carbohydrate counting, glycemic index/load considerations, and portion control.

3. Carbohydrate Quality: Not all carbohydrates are made equally. While reducing the intake of refined carbs and added sugars, placing an emphasis on whole grains, fruits, vegetables, and legumes,sources high in fiber, vitamins, and minerals can help stabilize blood glucose levels and encourage satiety.

4. Protein and Fat Considerations: Including sources of lean protein and healthy fats, including those in fish, avocados, nuts, and seeds, can improve lipid profiles, increase satiety, and help with weight management without having a negative impact on glycemic control.

5. The Stress of Nutrient Density Nutrient-dense foods, which include vital vitamins, minerals, and

antioxidants without being overly caloric or sweetened, are crucial, according to evidence-based nutrition. Accepting a wide range of nutrient-dense foods improves general health and lowers the chance of nutrient deficits.

6. Measuring and Adaptation: People with diabetes can evaluate the success of their dietary interventions and make required modifications in conjunction with healthcare providers by routinely measuring their blood glucose levels, lipid profiles, and other metabolic markers.

Possibilities and Difficulties

There are still a number of obstacles in the way of evidence-based nutrition in the management of diabetes. Effective implementation of evidence-based nutritional treatments is hampered by socioeconomic differences, cultural dietary practices, inconsistent dietary guidelines, and limited access to healthy foods.

However, there are unheard-of chances to overcome these obstacles and enable people with diabetes to make knowledgeable dietary decisions in line with evidence-based guidelines, thanks to advancements in digital health technologies, telemedicine, and nutrition education initiatives.

Chapter four

Practical Tips for Diabetes Management

Millions of people worldwide suffer from diabetes mellitus, a chronic metabolic illness marked by increased blood sugar levels. Particularly, type 2 diabetes is intimately associated with lifestyle choices like food, exercise, and general health practices. Maintaining a healthy lifestyle and engaging in regular exercise are essential to managing and preventing diabetes. This thorough guide will cover the importance of lifestyle modifications and exercise in managing diabetes, along with helpful hints for incorporating these activities into your everyday routine.

1. Recognize your situation.

When it comes to treating diabetes, information truly is power. Spend some time learning about the many forms of diabetes, their effects on the body, and any possible consequences. You can make more educated decisions regarding your health and available treatments if you have a clear understanding of your situation.

2. Cooperate closely with your medical staff.

You can properly manage your diabetes with the support of your healthcare team, which includes your doctor, dietitian, and diabetes educator. Create a customized diabetes management plan with them that takes into account your tastes, way of life, and health objectives.

3. Consistently check your blood sugar levels.

It's critical to routinely check your blood sugar levels if you have diabetes. With a blood glucose meter, record your readings and store them in a diary or mobile app. By keeping an eye on your blood sugar levels, you can spot patterns and trends and modify your treatment strategy accordingly.

4. Adhere to a nutritional plan.

Healthy, well-balanced diet is important for controlling diabetes. Consume a range of foods more of nutrients, such as whole grains, fruits, vegetables, lean meats, and healthy fats. Refined carbs, bad fats, and sugary meals should be consumed in moderation as they might elevate blood sugar levels.

5. Regulate the Size of the Portion

Maintaining a healthy weight and controlling blood sugar levels both depend on meal sizes. To determine the proper portion sizes for various foods, use measuring cups, spoons, or visual cues. A large amount of any food, especially one high in carbohydrates, should be avoided, as this can cause blood sugar levels to rise.

6. Recognize carbohydrates

Since carbohydrates have the most effect on blood sugar levels, it's critical to properly check your carbohydrate intake. Select complex carbs that have a low glycemic index, like those found in whole grains, legumes, and non-starchy vegetables. These foods digest more slowly and raise blood sugar levels gradually.

7. Continue to move

Engaging in regular physical activity helps to improve general health and manage diabetes. Try to get in at least 150 minutes a week of moderate-to-intense aerobic activity, such as swimming, cycling, or brisk walking. Incorporate strength training activities twice a week or more to increase insulin sensitivity and muscle mass.

8. Control your stress.

Stress can have an impact on blood sugar levels and increase the difficulty of managing diabetes. Use stress-reduction methods to help you unwind and preserve your emotional health, such as yoga, tai chi, meditation, or deep breathing. Seek out constructive ways to decompress, such as time spent with family and friends, hobbies, or artistic endeavors.

9. Get enough rest.For the treatment of diabetes and general health, getting enough sleep is crucial. For your body to heal and regenerate, try to get 7 to 8 hours of sleep per night. To encourage improved sleep quality, set up a consistent sleep schedule, establish a calming nighttime ritual, and reduce distractions in your sleeping surroundings.

10. Drink plenty of water.It's critical for diabetics to drink lots of water in order to stay hydrated and preserve good health. Try to drink 8 to 10 glasses of water and more if you live in a hot area or are physically active each day. Reduce the amount of alcohol and sugar-filled drinks you consume, as they can dehydrate you and alter your blood sugar levels.

11. Adhere to the prescription drug regimen.

Follow your doctor's instructions to the letter if you are provided medication to control your diabetes. Do not skip or increase dosages without first talking to your doctor; instead, adhere to the suggested timing and dosage. Discuss any worries you may have or

any adverse effects you may be experiencing right
away with your healthcare provider.

12. Remain upbeat and tenacious.

Diabetes can be difficult to manage, but you can
greatly improve your chances of success by keeping
a good outlook and persevering through your
symptoms. No matter how small, acknowledge your
accomplishments and don't let failures depress you.
Keep in mind that managing your diabetes is a
lifetime pp

Chapter five

Exercise and Lifestyle Factors

Millions of people worldwide suffer from diabetes mellitus, a chronic metabolic illness marked by increased blood sugar levels. Particularly, type 2 diabetes is intimately associated with lifestyle choices like food, exercise, and general health practices. Maintaining a healthy lifestyle and engaging in regular exercise are essential to managing and preventing diabetes. This thorough guide will cover the importance of lifestyle modifications and exercise in managing diabetes, along with helpful hints for incorporating these activities into your everyday routine.

Comprehending Diabetes and Physical Activity

Diabetes arises from insufficient insulin production or inefficient insulin utilization by the body. Insulin is a hormone that facilitates the uptake of glucose into cells for energy production and helps control blood sugar levels.

For a number of reasons, regular exercise is essential to managing diabetes:

1. Increased Insulin Sensitivity: Exercise makes your body more insulin sensitive, which enables cells to absorb glucose and react to insulin more effectively.

2. Blood Sugar Regulation: Even in the absence of insulin, physical exercise promotes the muscles' ability to absorb glucose for energy, which lowers blood sugar levels.

3. Weight Management: Losing or maintaining weight is facilitated by exercise, and this is crucial for diabetes management because being overweight can lead to insulin resistance and high blood sugar.

4. Cardiovascular Health: Diabetes raises the chance of stroke and heart disease. By lowering blood pressure and cholesterol and boosting

circulation, regular exercise enhances cardiovascular health.

Exercise styles for managing diabetes

There are three primary forms of exercise that people with diabetes can include in their daily regimen:

1. Aerobic Exercise: Also referred to as cardiovascular exercise, aerobic exercises raise heart and breathing rates. Some of these exercises are walking, jogging, cycling, swimming, and dancing. Try to get in at least 150 minutes a week, spread across multiple days, of moderate-intensity aerobic exercise.

2. Strength Training: To increase muscle strength and endurance, resistance or strength training exercises are performed with weights, resistance bands, or body weight. Include strength training activities that focus on your major muscle groups, including your arms, legs, back, chest, and core, at least twice a week.

3. Flexibility and Balance Exercises: While balance exercises, particularly for older people with diabetes, help reduce falls, stretching exercises help increase range of motion and flexibility. As part of your general fitness regimen, incorporate flexibility

and balancing exercises. Concentrate on stretching the main muscle groups and executing balance-enhancing motions.

4. Getting Enough Sleep: Getting enough sleep is crucial for managing diabetes and general health. To encourage better sleep quality, set a consistent sleep schedule, establish a calming bedtime routine, and aim for 7-8 hours of restful sleep each night.

5. Consistent observation and adherence to medication: Follow your doctor's instructions to frequently check your blood sugar levels and take your diabetic pills or insulin as prescribed. Note any symptoms or changes in your condition, as well as your prescription dosages and blood sugar levels.

Practical Tips for Incorporating Exercise and Lifestyle Factors into Diabetes Management

1. Set realistic goals: Gradually raise the intensity, duration, and frequency of your exercise and lifestyle improvements from tiny, doable starting points. Honor your accomplishments and practice self-compassion.

2. Find workouts and physical activities you enjoy. You are more likely to maintain long-term commitments to physical activities and workouts that you enjoy. Try out a variety of exercises to see what suits you the best: group fitness courses, walking, swimming, cycling, dancing, or any combination of these.

3. Plan Regular Exercise Sessions: Include exercise in your daily or weekly plan and treat it as a crucial appointment. Even on hectic days, strive for consistency and prioritize getting some exercise.

4. Mix It Up: Add a variety of aerobic, strength training, flexibility, and balancing activities to your workout regimen to keep it fresh and engaging. This increases overall fitness and targets various muscle areas, in addition to preventing boredom.

5. Include family and friends: Working out with people can make it more motivating and pleasurable. Ask your loved ones, friends, or coworkers to accompany you on your walks, exercises, or fitness courses. Encourage one another to lead wholesome lives.

6. Refuel Your Body and Stay Hydrated: To stay hydrated, drink lots of water prior to, during, and after exercise. Before working out, fuel your body with a balanced lunch or snack that includes both protein and carbs to avoid low blood sugar.

7. Listen to Your Body: Observe how exercise makes your body feel both during and after exercise. You should cease exercising and see your doctor if you feel any pain, discomfort, or strange symptoms.

8. Be Ready for Changes: Managing diabetes calls for adaptability to alterations in schedule, surroundings, or health. Prepare to modify your lifestyle and workout routines as necessary, and ask for help when you need it.

Chapter six

Monitoring and Adjusting

One of the most important aspects of managing diabetes is diet. For people with diabetes, maintaining weight, managing blood sugar levels, and lowering the risk of complications all depend on closely observing and modifying their diet. In this thorough book, we will examine the fundamentals of monitoring and modifying food in the management of diabetes, along with useful advice and techniques for maximizing nutrition and improving health outcomes.

Knowing About Diet and Diabetes

Elevated blood sugar levels are a hallmark of diabetes, a metabolic condition caused by either inadequate insulin synthesis or impaired insulin activity. The hormone insulin, which the pancreas produces, aids in the uptake of glucose by cells for energy and hence helps control blood sugar levels. The nutrition we consume has a direct impact on our blood sugar levels; thus, controlling our diet is essential to the treatment of diabetes. People with diabetes can better control their blood sugar levels and enhance their general health by keeping an eye on and making adjustments to their diet.Keeping an eye on blood sugar levelsFor people with diabetes, it's critical to regularly check blood sugar levels in order to evaluate the effects of food choices on glucose levels and make any required adjustments. There are numerous ways to keep an eye on your blood sugar levels, such as:

1. Self-Monitoring of Blood Glucose (SMBG): By pricking a fingertip and putting a drop of blood on a test strip, people can use a blood glucose meter at home to assess their blood sugar levels. Blood sugar levels can be monitored using SMBG before and after meals, as well as at other times of the day.

2. Continuous Glucose Monitoring (CGM): CGM devices continuously check blood sugar levels day and night using sensors that are implanted beneath the skin. Real-time glucose measurements and trends are provided by CGM, enabling more

thorough food and insulin medication monitoring and adjustments.

Important Dietary Guidelines for the Management of Diabetes

When tracking and modifying their dietary habits, people with diabetes should take into account the following important guidelines:

1. Carbohydrate Management: Since carbohydrates have the biggest effect on blood sugar levels, controlling carbohydrates is essential to the treatment of diabetes. Controlling the amount of carbs consumed and selecting low-GI carbohydrates will help maintain blood sugar stability and avoid spikes and crashes.

2. Portion Control: Achieving and maintaining a healthy weight, as well as controlling blood sugar levels, depend on portion sizes. Using measuring cups, spoons, or visual signals to measure quantities can help people control how much food they eat and avoid overindulgence.

3. Balanced Nutrition: For both general health and the management of diabetes, a diet rich in a range of nutrient-dense foods must be balanced. To supply vital nutrients and encourage fullness, concentrate on adding fruits, vegetables, whole grains, lean meats, and healthy fats to meals and snacks.

4. Meal Timing and Distribution: You may help stabilize blood sugar levels and avoid post-meal rises by distributing your daily carbohydrate consumption equally throughout the day and combining it with foods high in protein and fiber. To maintain steady energy levels and stave off hunger, aim for three well-balanced meals a day, plus snacks as needed.

Useful Advice for Tracking and Modifying Diets in the Management of Diabetes

1. Keep a food journal: By tracking food intake, portion sizes, and blood sugar levels with a food journal or a smartphone app, people can spot patterns and trends in their diet and make well-informed changes.

2. Regularly Check Blood Sugar Levels: Information from routine blood sugar checks before

and after meals, as well as at other times during the day, is helpful in modifying insulin medication and diet as necessary.

3. Recognize Carbohydrate Counts: Acquire the skill of interpreting food labels and calculating the carbohydrate contents of various foods and portion sizes. When arranging meals and snacks, consider the amount of each component and the amount of carbohydrates.

4. Select low-glycemic-index foods: Choose low-glycemic carbohydrates, which digest more slowly and don't raise blood sugar levels. Examples of these include whole grains, legumes, fruits, and non-starchy vegetables.

5. Play Around with Meal Scheduling and Composition: Examine various meal scheduling techniques, such as consuming smaller, more frequent meals or distributing snacks and meals equally throughout the day, to see the effects on hunger and blood sugar levels.

6. Track Blood Sugar Reactions After Meals: Observe how various foods and meals impact your

blood sugar levels after eating. To achieve the best post-meal glucose control, experiment with meal timing, content, and portion sizes.

7. Seek Advice from a Registered Dietitian: To create a customized meal plan that meets your unique requirements, preferences, and health objectives, speak with a registered dietitian who specializes in diabetes treatment. A dietitian can offer advice on meal planning, portion control, and label reading, in addition to managing carbohydrates.

8. Hydrated: To develop general health and stay hydrated, drink lots of water all through the day. Limit alcohol and sugary drinks, as they can raise blood sugar levels and cause dehydration.

Changing My Diet Depending on My Blood Sugar Levels

People with diabetes may need to modify their diets in order to better control their blood sugar levels, based on dietary observations and blood sugar measurements. The following are some methods for modifying a diet in response to blood sugar readings:

1. Modify Portion Sizes: Depending on blood sugar levels and energy requirements, modify the portion sizes of foods high in carbohydrates. To help lower blood sugar levels, think about reducing portion sizes or selecting lower-carbohydrate options.

2. Select Healthier Options: To help regulate blood sugar levels, swap out high-glycemic items for lower-glycemic ones. For instance, pick sweet potatoes over white potatoes or full-grain bread in place of white bread.

3. Balance Macronutrients: To support stable blood sugar levels and long-lasting energy, make sure meals and snacks include a reasonable proportion of protein, carbs, and healthy fats.

4. Watch timing and composition: To avoid blood sugar swings, keep an eye on the times and contents of meals and snacks. Make any necessary adjustments. Try out various meal combinations and scheduling techniques to see what suits you the best.5. Remain Consistent: To help control blood sugar levels and minimize significant swings, be consistent with meal times, portion amounts, and food selections.

Conclusion

Diet has a crucial role in determining health outcomes and quality of life in the complicated world of diabetes care. The multitude of dietary guidelines makes it necessary to dispel misunderstandings and adopt evidence-based nutrition habits that are specific to the requirements of people with diabetes. Through our investigation, we have uncovered the essential ideas that support sensible dietary control and debunked widespread myths that could impede advancement.

Gaining a thorough understanding of the complex intcraction between diet and the metabolic complexities of diabetes is the first step towards optimum diabetic management. Contrary to common assumptions, eating too much sugar is not the only cause of diabetes. Instead, it is a complex disorder impacted by a wide range of elements, such as environmental triggers, lifestyle choices, and heredity. Understanding that diabetes is a complex condition, people can control their diets more comprehensively than just cutting back on sugar.We dispel the idea of a one-size-fits-all nutritional prescription by dispelling myths about diabetes and diet. Diabetes can take many different forms, and each one requires a nutritional strategy that is specific to the needs and tastes of the individual. Some people may benefit from carbohydrate restriction, but others might do better on a balanced diet that prioritizes whole grains, fruits, and vegetables. People can develop long-term adherence and metabolic health by adopting sustainable eating patterns that include dietary diversity and customization.

In order to effectively control diabetes, evidence-based nutrition emphasizes the development of mindful eating practices that go beyond simple calorie restriction. By teaching people to recognize their own signals of hunger and fullness, mindful eating helps people develop a stronger bond with food and increase their level of dietary satisfaction. People can develop a better relationship with food and break free from the guilt and deprivation that are frequently connected to dietary restrictions by engaging in mindful eating practices.

The glycemic index stands out among the plethora

of dietary guidelines as a useful tool for selecting foods and achieving optimal glycemic management. It's a common misconception that all carbohydrates are equal. By giving information about how different foods affect blood sugar levels, the glycemic index enables people to make decisions that support stable glycemic management. People can lessen the chance of hyperglycemia and postprandial glucose excursions by making low-GI foods their first priority.

The Mediterranean diet is a shining example of nutritional excellence in the field of evidence-based nutrition, and it has several health advantages for people with diabetes. The Mediterranean diet, which is based on a diverse range of whole grains, legumes, fruits, vegetables, and healthy fats, is the perfect example of how flavor and nutrition can work together. It has numerous cardiometabolic benefits, including enhanced glycemic control, lipid profiles, and cardiovascular health, because of its concentration in plant-based foods, lean proteins, and olive oil. People who adopt the Mediterranean diet's tenets can go on a culinary adventure that satisfies their physical, mental, and spiritual needs. The value of individualized nutrition becomes clear as we make our way through the maze of dietary recommendations as a guiding principle for managing diabetes. Personalized nutrition adjusts dietary interventions to match each person's goals and health status, taking into account their specific needs and preferences. By means of thorough nutritional evaluations and continuous assistance, people can set out on a revolutionary path towards optimum well-being, equipped with the understanding and authority to make knowledgeable food decisions.

When it comes to managing diabetes, the path to optimal health goes beyond food changes and includes lifestyle adjustments that support overall health. The cornerstones of comprehensive diabetes treatment are medication adherence, physical activity, stress management, and good sleep hygiene. People can build a strong foundation for long-term health and vitality by combining lifestyle changes with an evidence-based diet.

As the conversation on nutrition's role in managing diabetes draws to an end, it serves as a reminder of how transformative nutrition can be in determining health outcomes and improving quality of life. People can confidently manage their diabetes by using evidence-based nutrition as a lens, giving them the information and power to adopt a nutritional paradigm that is founded on science, compassion, and delicious food. We are paving the road for a better future where people with diabetes may thrive and flourish, enabled by the transforming potential of evidence-based nutrition, by dispelling myths, embracing evidence, and cultivating an inclusive culture.

.